HOT

Sexy, DIRTY,

SEX TIPS

A Sexual Self Help Book

Written By Miss MiMi Jeune

HOT *Sexy*, DIRTY, SEX TIPS

A Sexual Self Help Book

Written By Miss MiMi Jeune

To the Reader,

 I think we should all be having the sex we want, and wanting the sex we have! I dedicate this book to all people that enjoy sex and want to have more of it!

Wishing you All the Best in Life, Love & Sex

Truly,

Miss MiMi

Contents

Introduction

I love sex! I know I'm not alone. Sex is a part of life. Sexual chemistry still can't be explained why we are attracted to certain people sexually. But there is a sexual chemistry that we encounter when someone arouses us. Sexual Chemistry can be taken to another level if two lovers are compatible. You can discover how sexually compatible you are by having an honest discussion about what you expect and desire sexually. I talk about sex all the time, even before I started giving tips on the radio. I think it's a natural discussion to have with those you care about. There should be no shame associated with your sexual preference. I believe there is no sexual ideal; there are gender roles but my motto! "If you like it I love it!" If we repress our sexual needs or feel judged because of our sexual desires we can become secretive about our desires and develop a secret sexual compulsion that may make you feel guilty. I encourage my listeners and readers to listen to their partners' needs and wants and to express their own. It's important that we talk about what we expect or desire sexually, if lovers aren't sexually compatible it could determine how long they will be together. The best way to find out what your lover is into is to ask. I have the hottest tips to help you "Nut Up or Shut up!" Read on for my HOT *Sexy, Dirty, Sex* **TIPS.**

Chapter 1: The Rules, Sex Safe, Unprotected Sex

"Oh me so horny! me love you long time!"

Sex is a natural part of life! It's nothing to be ashamed of. We all need to experiment sexually. We need to discover our sexual needs and reach our sexual wants. Sex is a powerful thing and what you don't know about sex and your lovers' sexual history can kill you. I have a lot of **HOT TIPS** in this book, but I have to address the reality of sex and the issues that can arise once you become sexually active. Safe and healthy sex should be the goal no one wants to risk a moment of pleasure for a lifetime of pain. Safe sex is a must. We all should be aware of the dangers of unprotected sex. Sexually transmitted Diseases (STD's) are still being spread. Unplanned parenthood is still an issue. We need to be more sexually aware and no longer spread a message of shame. Sex is good for you. Many instances sex is something you have to experience to understand. There are Rules to having healthy sex.

Read on for **HOT** *Sexy, Dirty, Sex* **TIPS.**

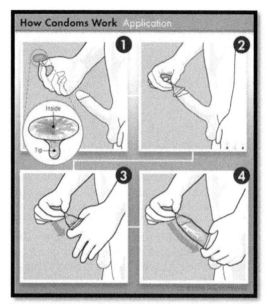

How to put on a condom

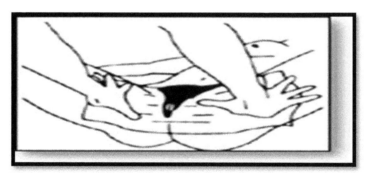

How to use a dental dam

HOT *Sexy*, `Dirty` TIPS:
The Rules, Sex Safe, Unprotected Sex

4 HOT TIPS for Safe Sex

1. Get to know your partner! Try not to have random sex with everyone you meet. If there is a sexual chemistry avoid having sex on the first date. It gives you something to look forward to. Giving it all up on the first date diminishes the attraction. You can't trust everything someone tells you, most of the time people tell you only what they want you to know. A one-night stand is a choice you make, there is no Sex Police to arrest you for "Reckless Fucking" Sex is a personal choice that has consequences. There are no sexual mistakes.

2. If you are sexually active doing anything sexual you need to use protection. Oral sex is a form of sex; flavored condoms for sucking dick or Dental dams can be used when eating pussy or ass.

HOT TIP: Create a Dental Dam by cutting a flavored condom in half and using it flavored side facing up.

3. Buy and use condoms. Size does matter, make sure you buy the correct size condoms. If your condom fits tight or only covers half your penis then you need to get a bigger size. Wearing a tight ass condom defeats the purpose of having safe sex. If your condom fits loose and slips off then you need a smaller size. If you don't know how to put a condom on, practice on a banana. I have met grown men and women that don't know how to properly put on a condom, if you never learned then you need practice.

4. Carry more than one condom, and ladies should carry condoms. Some women think they look easy or sleazy if they carry a condom. There is nothing cute about ignorance. A real woman that knows what she wants carries a condom. All women should carry a condom and have protected sex. There are even female condoms so there is no excuse not to have safe sex. Don't even let a dick touch or rub your pussy without a condom on. Many STD's are spread through contact.

HOT *Sexy, Dirty, Sex* **TIPS** *A sexual Self Help book*

Chapter 2: Mind Sex, Masturbation, Sensual Touch

"I was just thinking about you last night. It was a wet dream."

Your thoughts can bring you to an Orgasm! You can touch yourself until you reach an Orgasm, We can touch each other until we reach an Orgasm. Masturbation is OK!

Masturbation and thoughts of your lover can be very intense and sexually satisfying. Masturbation is the first step in discovering what you like and need sexually. It helps you explore your sexual needs and makes you feel comfortable sharing and expressing yourself sexually. Masturbation is a form of self love; it can build up your sexual confidence allowing you to express yourself sexually. We should never be ashamed of our own sexual self discovery! Sex is a natural part of life.

Dirty Thoughts, Masturbation, Sensual massage are all ways to explore yourself and your lover. Read on for my HOT *Sexy,* Dirty, *Sex* TIPS.

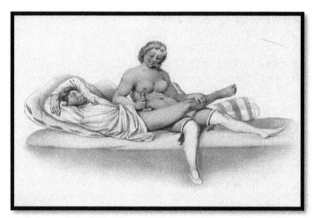

Gustav Klimt's "A Young Woman Masturbating" (1916).

HOT *Sexy*, Dirty TIPS :
Dirty Thoughts

We can visualize and manifest the sex we want! A Wet Dream, or recalling the hot sex that you had the night before are all ways to have Mind Sex and keep yourself aroused until you see your lover again. Not in a relationship, well sexy thoughts are a good way to keep sexiness in your life, think about how hot and intense it will be when you do meet a new lover, imagine how great the sex will be.

It's *Sexy* to share Dirty Thoughts. Tell your lover how you thought about the great sex, or an intimate moment that you shared. Tell them how you became hot all over again. Tell them that one thing they do that drives you wild. Your lover will love you for this! Sharing Dirty thoughts helps your lover know when they hit the spots.

HOT *Sexy*, Dirty TIPS :
Dirty Thoughts

LADIES:

We can manifest the Great Sex we want!
Concentrate on the Hot, Wet, Tight, and
Goodness of your untouched pussy. Think about
how much your lover will appreciate that you
have waited for them. Then try to visualize the
lover of your dreams touching you and making
you cum. If you are in a relationship concentrate
on the Best sex you have had, re-create the
moment in your mind, share your thoughts with
your lover tell your lover how you want to be
touched.

MEN:

Think about the passion that's building inside
you and how hard and pleasing you will be to
your lover. Think about holding you're cum back
until you explode.   Recall times when you really
pleased a lover and think about how you felt and
how your lover looked and acted afterwards.
Men are very visual they are more easily aroused
by thinking about Sex. Men tell your lover when
you have sexy thoughts about them; it's a
reassuring turn on.

HOT *Sexy*, Dirty TIPS:
Sensual Touch
Sensual Touch or massage is a *Sexy* way to make your partner more receptive to your sexual advances. If your lover is frigid or not easily aroused, then sensual massage will break the ice. There is something soothing and healing about sensual touch that calms a nervous lover.

HOT TIP for an Apprehensive lover: Just tell them you want to give them a massage, nothing more. Men and Women both can become frigid at times, not wanting sex due to a number of things. Reassurance is key let your lover know you are willing to wait, but you would like to relax them. Offering a full body massage or a foot rub is a great way to break the ice and bond with your lover.

Rubbing a naked body with warm oil and smooth strokes is *Sexy* relaxing and arousing. You can start with a foot massage and advance to a full body massage. Gently rubbing and caressing your lovers' body or feet can seem like a lot of work but the payoff is worth it once you see how aroused your lover has become. Sensual Massage can soothe the most frigid lover. Focusing on your lover, touching and caressing their body you can learn all the hot spots. Sensual massage regularly is a bonding experience for lovers; it makes you feel very comfortable with one another. Touching your lovers' entire body creates a deep bond. If you are looking to take your sex life to the next level add massage as part of your regular routine.

HOT *Sexy*, `Dirty` TIPS :
Sensual Touch

Something `DIRTY` to do while exploring Sensual Touch. Massage the private parts!

LADIES: Don't be afraid to massage the penis and balls. You would be surprised how a simple Dick and Balls massage will have your man moaning, and it's healthy for his prostate gland. You can make a man have an intense orgasm with a massage while you give them head. This before sex can make your man last longer. Don't forget to treat your man to a full body massage and foot rub. After a long day this can release all the tension and help him relax.

HOT TIP Pay attention to the area between the balls and the ass, it's very sensitive you should rub the area while giving him a dick massage or giving head.

MEN: All ladies love a good foot massage and a body rub. A short 15 minute body rub can help her relax and it shows you care. Don't neglect her most private parts they love massage as well. You can gently massage a woman's breasts. A leg thigh and butt massage can be great. Men can also massage during sex by rubbing the breasts when she is on top. In missionary you can grab and lift the ass while you fuck. It takes a little more concentration but its well worth the extra efforts when you use your hands.

HOT *Sexy*, Dirty TIPS:
Masturbation:

Most people are scared to admit that they masturbate. Self pleasure or masturbation is a powerful tool to learn what pleases you. I believe everyone should masturbate its part of building sexual confidence and it's a form of self love. Self Love is important through masturbation we learn how we like to be touched. This helps someone with little or no sexual experience guide a lover around erogenous areas. You can have some incredible orgasms by yourself or through mutual masturbation. So touch yourself it feels good.

LADIES

A *Sexy* thing to do is don't be afraid to touch and look at yourself. Take a mirror and look at your pussy get to know it. There is nothing wrong or gross about looking and touching your pussy. Especially if you are sexually active, you need to know what's going on down there. Touching yourself is a good way to feel yourself. Think *Sexy* thoughts about yourself. Think about how good your pussy is, how sexy you are; think about your lover tasting and teasing your pussy. Self love is important. You need to love and appreciate yourself before someone else will.

HOT TIP: Find someplace that is comfortable and private lie down naked and rub your hands around the sensitive parts of your body, breasts, stomach, inner thighs. Gently touch your vagina with your fingers, find your clit and rub in a circular motion. Rub and touch your clit with 1 or 2 fingers until you feel you are reaching a climax. If you want to explore further you can also try this with a vibrating sex toy placed directly on the clit until you cum. You can reach a great orgasm by yourself or with sex toys.

HOT Sexy, Dirty TIPS:
Masturbation:

MEN:

All men should masturbate. Masturbation can be great practice until you get the real thing. Your penis gets hard and you ejaculate. Masturbation can build up stamina and make you last longer. To make sure you have an incredible masturbation experience use lubricant and visual aids like Porn and Sexy magazines. Men take a mirror and look and touch your dick. It's important to know how your dick looks hard and soft.

HOT TIP:
Find a private place that you won't be interrupted and think about things that arouse you while you gently stroke your penis. You can use lubrication for a realistic feel. Stroke your penis until you become hard and erect. Think about your lover or someone you would like to be with. Stroke your penis faster until you climax. Men can also use sex toys. There are a lot of masturbators that are shaped like vaginas and can be filled with lubrication for a realistic feel. Masturbation is a form of safe sex that allows you to practice, but it gets a little Messy.

DIRTY **TIPS** for *Masturbation:*

COUPLES OR MUTUAL MASTURBATION:
Although it can't get too DIRTY, Mutual Masturbation or watching each cum can be an amazing experience. Challenge each other, how long you can do it without having intercourse? Dry Humping is something DIRTY you can do while masturbating. Ladies feel how wet your pussy will get with your panties on while you grind your pussy on him. Men can cum with clothes on, see how long you can go without having intercourse. The sexual tension that is building can lead to some very intense sex. Many women enjoy mutual masturbation. It allows them to open up more and become more comfortable with their lover. It's a turn on if a man is excited by a woman pleasuring herself. You can also use masturbation after sex to re arouse your partner for more sex.

LADIES: A *Sexy* thing to do is grind your pussy
on him, let him feel the wetness through your panties. Give your lover a Hand job with lubrication and massage the boys! Ladies you can also masturbate yourself during sex, rub your clit while he is fucking you, to intensify sex!

Dirty TIP: A Foot job! You can do this by rubbing you feet with lotion or lubrication. Then place the soles of your feet on the sides of his dick and stoke like you're giving him a hand job. Jacking the penis off between the soles, or between the toes of both feet can make your man cum.

HOT *Sexy, Dirty, Sex TIPS A sexual Self Help book*

MEN:

A **HOT** thing to do is caress and finger the vagina or kiss and play with the breasts. You can also finger her ass, a lot of women won't take a dick in the ass, but a finger is ok. Make sure you use lubrication and gently rub around her asshole while slowly pushing the finger and gently grind the finger in the ass.

A *Sexy* thing to do is use a vibrator on her. Many women use sex toys alone and have intense orgasms. You can use a vibrator on the clit until she cums or to cause multiple orgasms. This can be very intense. A woman can anticipate her own touch but a lover can make the feeling more intense by taking control and making the orgasm more unexpected.

Mutual masturbation can be as satisfying as actual sex, but your hands may get a little DIRTY.

HOT *Sexy*, *Dirty*, *Sex* **TIPS** *A sexual Self Help book*

Chapter 3: Sexy Hygiene , Trimming the Happy Trail, Pissy Privates Prevention

"What's that Smell!?? Are those your Dirty underwear?? What's the white stuff on your penis??"

Those are some of phrases that you don't want to hear in the bedroom! Sexual Hygiene is so important for men and women who are sexually active or thinking about having sex. No one likes Pissy Privates. You always want to be clean and fresh just in case you have an unexpected sexual encounter. There are many factors that even the cleanest person can have a smelly moment. That's why it's so important to keep all your private parts and any area you think your lover wants to kiss or lick on clean! I have a few Tips to help you stay your freshest! Read on for my HOT *Sexy,* Dirty, *Sex* TIPS.

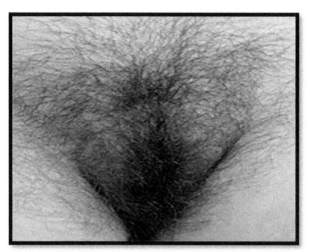

Hairy Pussy

HOT Sexy, Dirty TIPS:
Sexy HYGIENE

1. Good old soap and water is the number one way to stay fresh! Wash your ass. Use Deodorant. Clean your ears or anywhere you think someone will lick and kiss! Brush and floss! Clean your nails.

2. Sexy TIP: TRIM The Happy Trail
Men and Ladies trim your pubic hairs! Pubic hairs collect odor and smell DIRTY so keep them trim! Ladies SHAVE your legs and under arms! There is nothing attractive about a hairy woman.

3. BRUSH AND FLOSS and keep some breath mints if you think you will be kissing or having close contact.

4. LADIES & MEN: Keep your nails and feet clean. DIRTY hands and feet are very unattractive, and may make your lover think that you aren't clean.

5. LADIES & MEN: Clean underwear and socks. If you're planning on getting undressed if front of someone, don't wear dirty, ripped underwear! Just don't! It's DIRTY

HOT TIP: PISSY Private Prevention:
After a night of Drinking, Dinner, Dancing and a few trips to the bathroom. Please freshen up!

LADIES: Makes sure you wipe good, use baby wipes if you need to. Do a Breath check, and keep some mints or gum handy if you have been smoking and drinking.

MEN: Don't be afraid to wipe the penis off instead of your usual drip dry, after a few trips to the bathroom, the Penis can have a pissy smell.

Chapter 4: Oral Sex, Pussy Eating, Blow Jobs, Spit or Swallow

.

"RIGHT, THERE, PLEASE DON'T STOP!"... "Please suck it a little longer!"

This is what you want to hear if you're having Oral Sex! Oral Sex can be a incredible Orgasm when properly done, You can make your lover have intense orgasms or even multiple ones with the proper technique . Many women and men may never experience the joy of having an oral stimulated orgasm either because there lover hasn't learned how to properly do it or they aren't willing to do what it takes to make them cum. Even if it doesn't happen the first time, remember practice makes perfect!

TO SPIT OR TO SWALLOW that is the question! I say it's a matter preference and how you may feel at the moment! Many think this is a question only referring to the LADIES, but MEN have swallowing issues as well!

Read on for my HOT *Sexy,* Dirty, *Sex* TIPS to help you achieve that leg shaking orgasm you heard about.

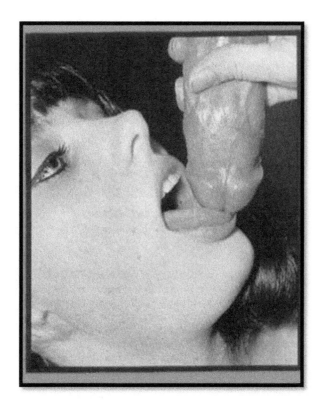

Vintage blow job

TO SPIT OR TO SWALLOW

MAN: "*I want you to swallow my cum!*"
WOMAN: "*NO, It's slimy, Yuk*", "*Tell me before you cum!*"

These are all the things you may hear and more if you ask a woman to suck the cum out of your dick! I am here to tell you its mind over matter! You can swallow some cum or at least act like you want to. Attitude is everything when it comes to the cum! Some may say "spitters are quitters", but just because you don't finish off doesn't make you bad at giving head. But you should try not to get so grossed out by cum, even if you get some in your mouth smile and spit it out. The *Sexiest* thing you can do is allow the cum to drip out of your mouth and wipe the rest off your face with the back of your hand. Make sure you tell him how sweet his dick tastes, and how you get a taste for him at times. But if your man wants you to swallow his cum you should at least try, it's not that bad and it's mostly water!

TO SPIT OR TO SWALLOW

MAN: *"Your Pussy is really wet."*
WOMAN: *"No that's your spit!"*

Yes men this means you! It may surprise you but not all men like to eat pussy! For every man that likes to eat it there is one who doesn't. Some of them have a tendency to salivate and because they don't want to "Swallow" they drool making the pussy very wet. There is nothing worse than half assed pussy eating. It can make your pussy seem wetter, but it doesn't always make it feel good! So if you are eating some Pussy "Suck it up" and "Swallow" as you lick, it may get a little messy, but there is a difference between a woman's cum and a man's sloppy drool.

HOT TIP: In case you do need to spit cum out or wipe your mouth keep a damp wash cloth nearby for quick clean up.

HOT *Sexy*, Dirty, *Sex* TIPS : PUSSY EATING

A Woman loves you to eat her pussy. Attitude is everything even if you are a beginner you can learn to love eating pussy. No woman likes a man that is squeamish about eating her pussy. A woman's pussy is a source of pride we need to know you want and love our pussy. A woman will over look a little dick if the head is good. Eating pussy or Cunnilingus is something ever man should master. Find out what makes your woman cum. Variety is key to the approach once a woman can sense your moves the intensity can be diminished. The *Sexiest* thing to do is vary the approach with pussy eating. A woman loves a man who eats her pussy with a hungry aggression, but we also appreciate the strong gentle approach, gripping a woman back towards you when you feel her trying to pull away.

A HOT TIP for *Pussy Eating*

Surprise pussy feasting is always good! When she least's expects it surprise her with oral sex! You should try to make a woman cum! We love you to eat our pussy. Stay in control, if you are about to make her cum grab her legs and hold her down, and eat her pussy until she can't take it.

A *Sexy*, TIP for *Pussy Eating*

Let her ride your face. Face riding lets her have control and it allows you to really please your lover. A good face fucking won't hurt you! It will give your woman something to remember. Super freaky sex makes a lasting memory! And any kind of pussy feasting lets a woman know you are into her and you appreciate her vagina

A Dirty TIP for *Pussy Eating*

Place her on all fours slightly open her legs and bury your face in her pussy, eat her pussy from the back stretching your tongue to her clit. Lick and Suck and Don't be scared to finish up with a ass licking!

TOP 5 *Blow Jobs* COMPLAINTS:

You know the drill start with a clean Dick and lick and kiss the head, lick down the dick and then put it in your mouth. Or you can put it in your mouth immediately, or Vice Versa. I have found there is more to giving a good blow job. Ladies attitude is everything when sucking a dick! The *Sexiest* thing you can do is suck a dick with a smile!

Even if you can't Deep Throat or if you're new to Blow Jobs, enthusiasm is key! I surveyed 200 women and these were the top 5 complaints about Blow Jobs.

1. Time, "How long" they have to do it.
2. Do I have to make you cum?
3. Do I have to swallow?
4. Do I have to lick your balls?
5. I can't suck it all, My jaws hurt!

Complaining leads to arguments! So instead of complaining or being against giving a blow job because you have a few objections; find a proactive solution. I know some men don't mind not getting a blow job. But there are very few that will turn down a good Blow Job! I feel a blow job is something a woman should try to master. There are times you may not be in the mood, but a man wants you to want his dick. It's a sense of pride to have a woman love and appreciate his dick. Even if you have been sucking the same dick for a while you should appreciate your dick and try to please it. It's very sensitive. There are a lot of ways to build up your dick sucking abilities. I think women need to take this seriously because for some men it can be a deal breaker. Even if you are a beginner, practice makes perfect.

TIPS for the TOP 5 *Blow job* COMPLAINTS:

1. **TIME?**: If time or how long you have to suck it is a issue then start to time yourself literally, either watch the clock or get a stop watch. Try to increase your time by 5 minutes every time. But just don't let the clock watching interfere with your finesse.

2. **Making Him Cum?** : OK this is a tuff one and just because you can't make him cum or ejaculate from a blow job doesn't mean you aren't good. Some men are harder than others. It's good to give it a try use your hands to work it along half sucking and half hand job does the trick.

3. **Swallow?**: No you don't have to swallow if you don't want to, but if he wants you to you should try at least once. A great way to get a around swallowing even if you have a mouth full of cum. I suggest letting the cum drip and drool out of your mouth and then wipe it off. If you don't want to touch the cum at all, just play with it a little and wipe it off.

4. **The Balls?**: OK some men don't believe in manscaping (trimming the pubic hairs) that can make the balls less appetizing, but if the droopiness or how they look is a turn off then just try to kiss them and lick them quickly. The balls are a part of the dick. There is really no way around this men like their whole dick touched

5. **It's too Big, It Won't Fit?**: If a gag reflex is part of the problem or you have a small mouth, then you need to have a juicy mouth and a fast hand! A gag reflex or a small mouth doesn't mean you can't suck a good dick! Your focus shouldn't be on deep throating, you will have to work at making your man appreciate your blow job abilities. Your juicy mouth can get the dick nice and wet and use your hand to jack the dick while you suck, kiss and lick the penis head. Yes you still can suck on the head and jack the penis

HOT *Sexy*, *Dirty*, *Sex* TIPS *A sexual Self Help book*

HOT Sexy, Dirty, & TIPS :
69, AND OTHER COMBO ORAL SEX MOVES!

A combo oral sex move can be an intense experience, the more we arouse each other the more we ravish each other! No taking turns here or arguing about who goes first, because the goal here is to please each other at the same time.

The 69 is a Sexy combo move can be an incredible sharing of oral sex, Woman on top or vice versa. It can be an intense orgasm because you are giving head at another angle many women find they can suck dick longer and stay in the moment more in a 69. Men tend to eat pussy longer as well, because they want you to continue sucking their dick. So if you are looking for longer or more Oral Sex then the combo moves are for you.

A Dirty combo move I like is do a 69 while lying on your side, this way it's easier to stimulate the ass, and play with the balls. Men also have deeper access to the pussy and the ass at the same time.

HOT TIP for Oral Sex is to use fruit or something flavored to make you really suck and swallow the cum. A strawberry or peach rubbed gently inside a pussy can make it taste sweet you can also add something sweet while you suck on his dick they have flavored edible lubrications that dissolve fast but leave flavor and make your mouth juicier while you suck his dick. It's all a matter of personal taste. Don't use something too messy, you don't want to use anything that will leave a residue or cause a big mess.

Sexy TIP for Oral sex is to change the sensation. Changing the temp is a pleasant surprise during a blow job or pussy eating. Suck on ice and immediately place your cold mouth on your lover and suck them until they warm up.

Chapter 5: The Vagina, Va-jay-jay, Pussy, Coochie

.

Pussy is power! It's a sexual fruit! It's both refreshing and life giving! Ladies the more we appreciate and know our vagina the more confident we become! We don't give as much credit as we should to the vagina, but it's nothing short of amazing! It's like a little machine, it's self pleasuring and self lubricating and it creates life with a little additive .

It can bring us so much pleasure. I encourage all women young and old to get to know their vagina on a personal level. Keep her happy and protect her! Give her that once a month break she needs to clean herself up and she is off and going once again. The vagina gives new meaning to the phrase " it takes a licking and keeps on ticking." Since the vagina is a muscle, the more you use it the better it gets! That's right so use it, it's like exercise for your insides. It's very precious so take good care of it you can't get another one, and who wants to go thru that designer vagina surgery for upgrades...seriously! Read on for my HOT *Sexy*, Dirty, *Sex* TIPS for the Va-Jay Jay!

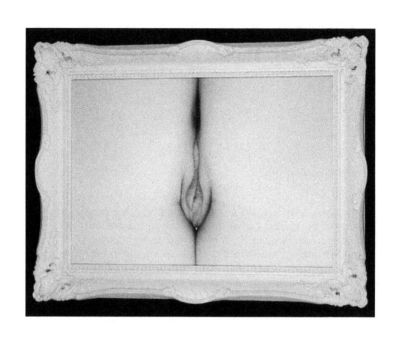

Pussy Eating

The pussy will surprise you! It has so many hot spots that with proper stimulation you can have amazing multiple orgasms through oral stimulation. You can start by gently start kissing down her body, if you are new to pussy eating and aren't that into it the *Sexiest* thing you can do is kiss a pussy. Start by gently kissing around the vagina area, then kiss the inside of the pussy gently insert your tongue and lick until you feel the clit at the tip of your tongue. The Clit is actually like a little penis . A *Sexy* thing to do is lightly suck and lick on the pussy. This will cause the clit to raise up and make is more sensitive to tongue stimulation. Lick the pussy and apply gentle pressure with your tongue until you feel it getting wet. Continue licking from the clit to the pussy hole you can speed up your tongue and apply a little pressure with your tongue until your lover cums.

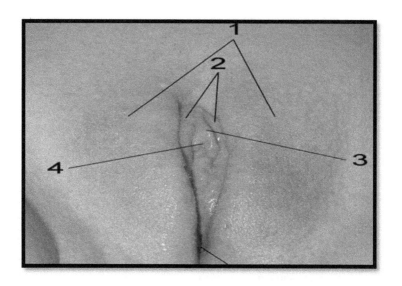

HOT Dirty TIP : **Pinch the Pussy!**

It may seem crazy but pinching the pussy is a different type of stimulation. Use the picture above to guide you. Gently squeeze on either side of the #1. It will gently raise up part 2, 3, 4. The clit has been compared to a small penis. When you Pinch the outside lips and gently try to grab the clit, you can actually jerk the clit! Do this by gently squeezing the outside of the pussy until you feel the clit from the outside. When you lightly grab or pinch the pussy you stimulate the sides of the clit. You can do this while you eat the pussy gently pinch the outsides of the pussy, this will gently raise the clit up, you can lick and suck the clit all at the same time. While you lick it apply a little pressure. Always remember never ruff with the pussy, when it comes to touch, gentle is better

Chapter 6: The Penis, Dick, One eyed Monster

The Penis has a mind of its own. Dicks come in all shapes and sizes we should love them all equally! Men if you give good head there are many women who will over look the size of a dick! A man actually needs sex, he has to ejaculate it's actually good for his health, it helps to flush out his prostate gland! We all want healthy men right! Another fact about the Dick, it that when a man is erect he is relaxed, yes its true, and it may seem like the other way around, but when the blood rushes to the penis it relaxes him! Keep this in mind when trying to satisfy your man or anyone else's! Instead of looking at it as a time consuming chore caress and appreciate the penis! Show some affection to his erection, even if it's hard all the time, don't push it away it gets like that for a reason, get to know it. It extends to greet you! You will always see eye to eye with a Penis if you show it some loving affection, the Penis won't let you down, and your man will love you for it! Read on for my HOT *Sexy,* Dirty. *Sex* TIPS

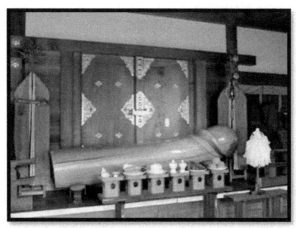

Penis Shrine in Japan

HOT *Sexy*, Dirty TIPS : *The Penis, Dick, and One eyed Monster*

Touch his Dick it's *Sexy*. A man's penis loves attention. It's a vulnerable area for a man, your man, will really appreciate you grabbing and holding his dick! It will relax him. One of the *Sexiest* things you can do is gently play with his dick and balls. When you are alone I suggest that you keep your hands on his dick as much as possible. If it sounds freaky it's because it is! If you are watching a movie grab his dick. It likes to be cuddled. If your man is angry it will help calm him down. If he doesn't want to be touched at the moment, don't take it personal , just try again at another time. But never stop trying to grab for his dick. The Penis loves attention.

Creativity, attention and enthusiasm are all KEY when getting dirty with your blow jobs. Men want their whole dick sucked. Sucking is also key, try to suck as hard as you can with as much of the dick in your mouth as possible. Be careful not to rub your teeth against the dick. Get into it you can make up for what you miss if you can't deep throat, if you suck his dick with a smile and tell him how sweet he tastes.

HOT TIPS FOR *a Curved dick :*

All Dicks are not created equal! The sizes and shapes vary. Some are large some are small, Some have curves, some Stand tall! A dick curved at the right angle can hit the g-spot! But if the dick curves in the wrong direction it can be a challenge! Ouch there is nothing worse than getting fucked with a curved dick at the wrong angle! Talk about digging you out! Instead of screaming it hurts stop. My first suggestion is see which way the dick curves. The trick with fucking a man with a curve dick is lifting up the same leg as the direction of the curve in the dick, you may have to position yourself at the angle of the dick. If the penis curves Upward it may be best to get on top and ride it or take it from the back.

Sucking a curved dick can be tricky as well! You have to suck it at the same angle it curves so you need to position yourself at the right or the left of the dick. If the Dick curves Upward you need to suck the dick in 69 position if you are having gagging problems.

HOT *Sexy.* Dirty TIPS : *The Penis, Dick, and One eyed Monster*

"How about a Dick Sandwich with a side of tossed salad"

HOT TIP
To make a Dick sandwich take both hands and grab underneath the balls gently pulling the balls on either side of the Dick Cupping the balls in your palms. Gently start to kiss and lick and suck the head of the dick while hold the balls gently near the top jacking the dick and sucking at the same time. Gently let the balls go. Deep Throat the dick as much as you can. Lick the balls and around the dick. Lick in between the balls and the asshole, if you want the "side of tossed salad" now go for it! (as long as his ass is clean and he will let you near that area) Then come back up for more dick sucking, deep throating as much as you can and jacking his dick until he comes.

A Dirty Tip: A Chocolate Dipped Dick topped with Whipped cream! It's *Sexy* to have something sweet with your dick. You can dip your dick in whatever you like, don't use a lot it can get messy and you don't want to leave residue. I like to use a spoon to lightly drizzle a small amount on the sides and rub it around. Use a little whipped cream on the sides and viola!

Sexy TIP : Use something cold. Different sensations are key in making Dick Sucking great. You can try hot and cold sensations with popsicles or ice. Changing the temp on your lover unexpectedly is very *Sexy*. Suck on a Popsicle or let an ice cube melt in your mouth before going down on your lover is an unexpected thrill. Suck him until his dick warms up.

THE BALLS:

One neglected area on a man is his balls! A *Sexy* tip is to grab and massage the balls. Also be careful not to pull the hair. In my dick sandwich I try to include the balls in the move. So it's very important that you play with them when you such his dick or give him a hand job. Some people say they are droopy or hairy, but get use to them they will be hanging around and they are a part of the dick!

Chapter 7 : Positions, Sexercise, Fucking

"Open your legs." Bend over." Put your legs in the air" Hit it from the back."

Positions are what you make them. There are so many variations and hot moves to try. Most of us never really get past the basic moves to challenge ourselves sexually. Arousal and Orgasms are powerful things that can make you have one impulsive instinct to immediately go into missionary position or the position that will make you cum the fastest. But faster is not always better when trying to have great sex. I suggest that we try to be more mindful and challenge ourselves to try some new moves or variations with our sexual positions. Sex can be so much fun when done properly. Sex is a form of exercise, you can burn 200 calories or more having a sex marathon! But we need to be less selfish and make sure that both of you are pleased during sex. Read on for my HOT *Sexy,* Dirty, *Sex* TIPS.

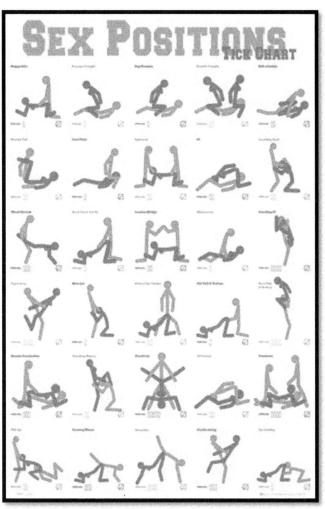

Sex positions chart

HOT *Sexy, Dirty, Sex* **TIPS** *A sexual Self Help book*

Sexy, Dirty TIPS **FOR** *Positions,*
Sexercise, Fucking

Having good sex is amazing. Sex is a stress relief.
Different sex positions offer different orgasms,
some are more intense than others. I surveyed
200 people asking the question: "What's your
favorite position?" Missionary was the 1#
position and Doggy style was in 2nd.

Yes we all love the missionary position and doggie
style but the *Sexiest* thing you can do is go through
the motions and create your own position, see how
far you can twist and turn without the dick pulling
out. It's almost like playing naked Twister. Sex
positions are great to explore and try something new.
You can have sex sitting, standing, leaning whatever
positions that works, then work it.

Some HOT TIPS for better sex :

LOCATION, LOCATION, LOCATION
If you always have sex in the same place, then switch
it up. This can make a good thing even better. Having
sex in other places outside the bedroom can be very
intense and *Sexy.*

CHALLENGING POSITION
You don't have to get a hernia, but you can try some
variations like standing and using the wall for balance.
Lifting one leg up or adding a pillow under your butt
for deeper penetration. Sex in a chair is a HOT
thing to do, try to grip the sides with your legs for
more control. Challenging positions can make you
both cum together.

SEX TOYS:

They have a lot of cock rings, vibrators and other sex toys on the market to enhance sex. There are sex wedges, swings, Leg holders and many other position enhancers to make the most of your sex. A vibrating cock ring is a small thing that can make sex amazing! Just get the right size, they can get stuck.

Sexy. Dirty TIPS FOR *Positions, Sexercise, Fucking*

LADIES: A Sexy thing to do is try something new and stay involved! If he is always on top make sure you are pumping back and lifting your legs up. If you normally ride the dick, then ride it backwards and play with his balls. Get more active during sex. Nobody likes to feel like they are doing all the work. Stay involved and tell him what works for you.

MEN: Try to control your cum as long as you can. Stopping and gradually letting your ejaculation build up will intensify your orgasm, and make you a considerate lover. Don't go so hard so fast unless your lover asks for it. No matter how excited you are gentle is always better. If you are too aggressive you may cum faster. You lover will let you know when to go faster The longer you delay to orgasm the more intense it is.

HOT *Sexy, Dirty, Sex* TIPS *A sexual Self Help book*

Chapter 8: Back Door ,Anal Sex, Getting it in the Ass

"Oh it hurts!".. ".No you can't touch my ass!"..."Please touch my ass"..."Oooh lick my ass!"....

Those are the mixed feelings associated with anal play. Some people hate it and are scared to try others, may try it and don't like it. Then you have those that love it! There are many people that are curious about anal stimulation.

There has been much debate about anal sex, but you can have an intense orgasm with any kind of anal stimulation when done properly it can cause body shaking orgasms. If you are completely against anal sex, it's understood there is some pain associated with it, but once you get past the pain, it can be a great experience for a couple that is exploring sex. Read on for my HOT *Sexy.* Dirty. *Sex* TIPS and don't forget the lubrication!

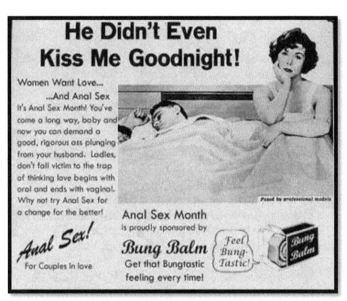

Vintage Anal sex Advertisement

Sexy, Dirty TIPS :*Back Door, Anal Sex*

Anal Stimulation can be great, but if you don't want to do it or if you are scared at all then I say don't do anything you aren't comfortable with. Anal sex does seem savage and DIRTY , but there can be some *Sexy* things about it. There are some rules it can be DIRTY so you want to play it safe and use a condom. I have Anal Sex Rules.

HOT TIPS Anal Sex Rules
1. Wash your ass. Anal sex usually involves anal licking. Make sure you and your partner Clean up before any type of DIRTY anal play .

2. Stay protected even long term relationships it best to stay protected. You are having sex in the ass, and it can get DIRTY . It has never been my experience but you can shit on a dick!

3. No DIRTY Double Dipping you should never let someone put a penis in your pussy after it comes out the ass, it can cause some problems. You will need to change condoms after anal sex

4. Lube, Lube,Lube! It's necessary; it could be a very painful experience without it! So lube up and when in doubt lube some more. Yes the condom does have lubrication but more is needed for the least painful experience.

HOT TIP For Anal: Silicon Based lubrication works best for anal sex! Water based lubes tend to dissolve faster. Silicon based lubrication lasts longer!

5. Make sure you have had a bowel movement. Anal sex is not something you do after dinner. You don't want to shit on the dick.

6. Warm it up! First start with some simple anal play before you try the intercourse. You can try lubricated fingers. You can try a butt plug or an anal vibrator. Anal play will make the asshole wet and aroused.

Sexy, Dirty TIP FOR Back Door, Anal Sex

ANAL PLAY

Anal play is very Sexy if you do it gently a finger in the ass during sex can cause an intense orgasm. If someone uses a dildo or fingers you in the ass in can make you cum. It will also help you if you are curious about anal sex. A Butt plug during sex can warm you up for anal sex.

BEGINNER ANAL

OK take a deep breath it will hurt a little but if you have decided to try anal sex, you can do it. Follow the rules so you won't have any Dirty accidents. Lay a towel down just in case. (Hey you are taking it in the ass!) There are a few beginner positions that will allow you the most control. You will need lubrication

TOP 4 ANAL POSITIONS

You can have anal positions in more than just doggy style.

Spooning is a great *Sexy* position that allows you to have control of how fast and hard you get it in the ass.

Getting on top may seem like a painful way, but this *Sexy* position allows you to have the most control, you can slowly sit on the dick gradually letting it slide in stopping when you need to but don't take it out too fast.

Missionary is a *Sexy* anal position, it's one of my favorite ways to get it in the ass. You would begin the same way you would have regular sex but instead you place the dick in the asshole and slowly pump until the dick is completely in.

Doggy Style is a HOT Dirty way to get it in the ass, but it may cause you to tighten up. It's not always the best way to do it. You need a lot of lubrication, try to lean back into the dick to prevent it from slipping out. The ass is not like the pussy if you are a beginner this is not the position for you.

ANAL INTERCOURSE if you think you are
ready for anal sex, then you should pick a position,
play it safe and give it a try. If it's your first time you
should use a lot of foreplay, massage, oral sex
whatever gets you the most aroused. Take it slow,
don't rush if you want to stop let your partner know.
No one should force you into any type of sex. Set some
rules before hand to let your partner know you have
limits. You can warm up during regular sex using a
dildo or fingering. A butt plug during sex can be
intense orgasm from double penetration.

When you are aroused and have a comfortable
position like **Spooning**; place the head of the
lubricated penis near the asshole. You should slowly
push back on to the dick until the head gets in. Once
the head gets in your partner should push back until
his dick is completely in the ass, don't pull it out or
stop abruptly, grind with the dick in the ass. Many
men cum fast, but don't pull it out fast, you could turn
your asshole inside out and it will be painful. But if
you take it slow and just breathe. When you pull it out
take it slow even a semi hard dick can hurt if you pull
it out to fast. Men need to be real easy when
approaching anal sex every woman doesn't respond in
the same way. You can learn to like anal sex and it will
give you some intense orgasms.

Chapter 9: Ménage Trios, 3Somes, Group Sex

This is a fantasy that many people WOMEN and MEN want to experience Ménage Trios; Two women and One man or vice versa. Swinging or Group sex parties are becoming more common. There are more "OPEN" relationships where "couples "are actively dating outside of their "committed" relationship. There are skeptics and it may not be your cup of tea, but don't close the idea completely off, until you hear your lovers view on it. No you may not be ready for some crazy "Swingers Party", but you may be open to trying a threesome, if not that's OK to, never feel pressure to try things sexually you are not that into! But if you are thinking about experimenting a *Sexy* thing to keep in mind, any kind of "Group Sex" is more about Sex not love! Read on for my HOT *Sexy*, Dirty, *Sex* TIPS.

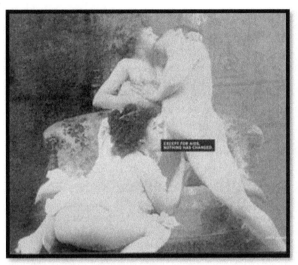

Vintage porn safe sex advertisement

HOT *Sexy, Dirty, Sex* TIPS *A sexual Self Help book*

HOT , *Sexy*, Dirty TIPS : *Ménage Trios, 3Somes, Group Sex*

A 3some or Ménage Trios can be something *Sexy* for you and your lover to experiment with. If you and your lover have decided to try some sort of group sex interaction then you must be really close and have a lot of trust. Always remember group sex encounters are only about sex. This can be a tricky situation if not approached properly. I have a 5 Hot *Sexy* TIPS if Group Sex is something you want to try.

HOT TIPS **Group Sex Rules**

1. It can be Dirty to have sex with someone you really don't know. Any type of group sex should be protected at all times.

2. Set some *Sexy* rules, if this is something new for you and your partner then you need to set some boundaries. I know it may seem weird, but you might not want your lover tongue kissing the jump off. If you are in a swinging situation you may not want your woman getting cum shots in the face.

3. Trust and honesty is the most important part in deciding to open your relationship. Decide on who picks the 3rd party, or if you are going to be in a swinging situation decide how you pick the couple together.

4. Try to be a pleasing lover you may not see this person again. It's *Sexy* to make the most of the situation.

5. No follow up, no sleepovers. Many times this is a onetime thing so decide as a couple if the 3rd party is someone you both want to keep in your life.

Chapter 10: Sexting, Sex Tapes, Computer love, Virtual Sex

Sex is on the internet and Social Networking is the new way to interact. Technology is so advanced that we now have real time video chats, people are having webcam sex and loving it! You can meet someone and learn what seems like a lot of information in a short amount of time through Social networking or dating website's. But be warned people only tell you what they want you to know. There are many success stories of people that have made great connections even marriage from internet rendezvous. We are more connected than ever, you can send impulsive instant messages and pictures documenting your every move and capturing your moments and feelings instantly! Virtual Sex is instanteous, safe and satisfying and addictive people are having webcam sex. This impulsive behavior has some downsides when you start to send personal information or naked pictures to your lovers. There is a sexting trend that people feel the need to send *Sexy*, messages that aren't met for everyone. I have some HOT TIPS for making the most of your Computer love. Read on for my HOT *Sexy*, Dirty, *Sex* TIPS.

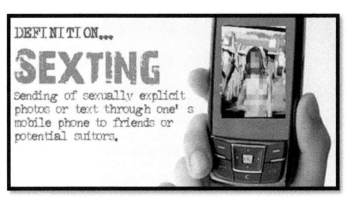

Anti Sexting advertisement

HOT , _Sexy_,, Dirty TIPS : Internet Dating

Internet dating and social networking are the new way to connect and meet. When you really think about it, there is really no difference from meeting a total stranger on the street. There are many success stories from internet dating and there is a dating site for just about anything you want to try online. I have some 5 Rules for Internet Dating success.

HOT TIPS Internet Dating

1. be as honest as you can. Don't post 5 year old pictures that look nothing like you currently. It's miss leading and wrong for ladies or men to post pictures that aren't current.

2. Don't fall into computer love before actually meeting someone. The internet makes dating multiple people easy! So don't get emotional about someone you really don't know, especially if you see them online a lot.

3. Only tell people what you want everyone to know. Don't put all your information out there. A brief summary and some interesting facts about yourself are OK. No need to put your address or area you live or work in. You wouldn't want to attract a stalker that knows all your moves.

4. Don't believe everything you read, people only tell you what they want you to know, you have to find the rest out. Don't be too impressed with pictures of cars or expensive items. The internet is an easy way to lie or exaggerate the truth

5. Beware of people that spend too much time online, unless they are a public person and have actual business online. You should steer clear of anyone spending 8 hours or more online. It makes you question there motive

HOT *Sexy,* Dirty, *Sex* TIPS
Tips FOR : Sexting,

Sexting or sending " *Sexy* "text messages or e-mails is a way some people are keeping in contact. The problem with these messages is that the messages that are met for that "special someone "are getting blasted to everyone. This has been a big problem with teenage sex. Many parents are reading messages and finding out their teenagers are sexual active. Deleted messages aren't even safe. Cheaters are being exposed by computer hacking lovers trying to uncover the truth. In many cases Sexting is not *Sexy,* and should be avoided! It's not something good to send if you aren't sure that the messages will be completely private.

I have 5 Sexting Rules, if you feel you can't avoid sending them.

5 HOT TIPS FOR **Sexting,**

1. No Drunk Texting, it can be an embarrassing situation answering questions about messages you don't remember sending. It's best to put your phone away if you get tempted to send messages once you get drunk.

2. Don't send "Major" news or something that should be said in person.

3. Proof read your texts especially if the info in the message is for a certain someone. With all the new smart phones is really easy to send a message to all your contacts.

4. Be Discreet! Even if this is your boo! You need to be careful not to say too much!

5. Texting has a curfew, avoid sending late night messages when possible, unless you are responding to someone immediately. It's not *Sexy* to send a text in the middle of the night, unless you know it's OK.

HOT *Sexy,* Dirty, *Sex* TIPS FOR: SEX TAPES

Sex Tapes seem to be the latest *Sexy* thing to do with your lover! There is nothing wrong with videotaping your lovemaking to watch yourselves in action, but there are some rules so the video doesn't end up as a must see! Or worse copied and sold as amateur porn! Many couples make videos for various reason either to mark a special moment like a honeymoon or a anniversary! But these types of video should be private and consensual unless both parties agree to release it for whatever reason. I have 5 Hot Tips for making a Sex Tape!

5 HOT TIPS For making a SEX TAPE :

1. **Consent!** Make sure both parties have agreed to make the video. There is nothing lower than taping a sex act with someone Man or Woman without consent. Make sure you trust the person you are making the sex tape with! Making a sex tape with a guy or girl you have only known for a short time is no good. You should have some type of bond unless you're a porn star, in that case make sure you get paid first before filming.

2. **Set the scene!** Make it good. Don't just tape some random sex act. LADIES : put on your *Sexiest lingerie* and sex it up for the camera! MEN : Put on some sexy undies. Light candles, whatever you like, it is your video!

3. **Get a camera!** Most Mini DV cameras are fine, try not to use a webcam, some give grainy footage, and that's not good when you want to watch the tape later.

4. **The Money Shot!** When filming make sure you pay attention to camera angles. If you switch positions you may have to switch the camera as well. There is no point of going through all the

motions only to find out your back was to the camera! So make sure the good parts are in clear view!

5. **Ownership!** You have to decide who keeps the tape! The manly thing to do is let the woman keep the sex tape! If you guys are together you can always hook up and watch the video together! But if you have anything at risk, or have any type of trust issues then you should watch the tape together and erase it together when you think the time is right.

HOT , Sexy,, Dirty TIPS FOR : Virtual Sex

Virtual sex is on the raise there are even social networks dedicated to virtual sex. It's safe, and private, and you can have some fantasies fulfilled by finding someone with mutual interests or that is willing to please you. It usually involves a chat some type of mutual masturbation via a web cam and a short chat afterward. There is some advanced virtual sex technology out there.

HOT Sexy, Dirty, Sex TIPS A sexual Self Help book

5HOT TIPS for Virtual Sex:

1. Find a partner for virtual sex using chat rooms, many people post up ads looking for virtual sex

2. Location: Yes even online you have to find a webcam chat place to meet on line. A virtual sex bar, or social network to meet up.

3.Chat about what your fantasies are.

4. Be descriptive about what's happening tell them how aroused you are or what you would do if they were actually there with you.

5. Don't get caught with your pants down. Make sure no one will walk in on you having sex online.

Acknowledgments

This book is about more than sex. It's about understanding we all need others to try and understand us our needs and wants. I believe the way to this understanding is by experience, trial and error, desire for improvement and manifestation. I live in love so I experience it daily in many forms. My immediate circle of people are all positive. I try to engage others when I sense a kindred spirit that holds the same values or some I could learn from. I could say I did it all by myself, but my life is nothing without people that see my value, support and encourage me. I want to thank all the people who encouraged me to be myself and live my dreams no matter what they are. PRICELESS! I want to Thank the following people for their support: My Mom for her encouragement without my dysfunctional but happy childhood none of this would be possible. DJ Whoo Kid who gave me an opportunity to run my mouth. I will always be grateful to you. The Gomez Brothers Gaby and Nels they are my brothers from another mother the synergy we share is amazing their vision and guidance is irreplaceable. I would also like to thank any haters or people whose condescending views are only their own reflection. Hate is the greatest form of love, because you care enough to think of me so much.

My mission when I started giving my Sex Tips was to encourage others to address the tuff sexual questions and preferences without being biased, there is no sexual ideal. I want to encourage people to challenge themselves sexually. I feel we should be able to say what we need without shame or fear of judgment. I want to speak directly to people that had pre conceived ideals about sex and challenge them to change that! I encourage people to listen to their lovers' needs and wants. I hope this book can be a tool

HOT *Sexy*, *Dirty*, *Sex* **TIPS** *A sexual Self Help book* for you to use to have the sex you want and want the sex you have.

I was told by a porn star friend of mine, I had the hottest sex tips around!! I give them out weekly on the radio. I can't take all the credit, yes I am a very sexually liberated person, I have done more than my fair share of experimenting. The Sex Tips I give are not solely my own they are a collection of what I have personally done or something someone that is close to me has shared. Please use them and enjoy! Be encouraged to build up your sexual self confidence by loving yourself first it will liberate all areas of your life.

ABOUT THE AUTHOR

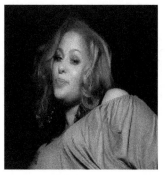

Miss MiMi is a radio personality, Sexpert, Author and so much more. You can listen to her host the Gomez Brothers| G-spot hour live on Sirius|XM Shade 45|XM 66 Saturday 7pm-8pm est. She gives Hot Sex Tips and advice about Sex and Love and creating a healthy balance in your life through self love. She has been a guest   relationship expert on many radio shows. She is renowned for her no nonsense and matter of fact approach to the subject matter.

She has spoken to 1000's of teens about the dangers and consequences of becoming sexually active. She is working on a book for Teens and their parents about sex.
Stay tuned into Miss MiMi she has many projects in the works.

Contact Miss MiMi

Sex Tips or Advice:
Call 347-223-5199
msmimigspot@gmail.com

Press or Bookings Contact:
Stephanie Carnegie :
thecarnegiegroup@gmail.com

RESOURCES

Planned Parenthood
http://www.plannedparenthood.org/

Aids and HIV Awareness
http://www.aids.org/
http://www.hhs.gov/aidsawarenessdays
http://www.marvelynbrown.com/

STD information
www.cdc.gov/STD

Teen Sex
www.talkingwithkids.org

Free Condoms
www.condomusa.com

Women's health awareness
www.nationalbreastcancer.org

Penis Health
www.prostatehealthguide.com

US Health Department
http://www.hhs.gov

Trojan Condoms
http://www.trojancondoms.com

PICTURE CREDITS

Picture Credits
Pages 7
Safe Sex Condom
How stuff works.com
Page 7
Sex   Vaginal
How stuff works.com
Page 18

Gustav Klimt's "A Young Woman Masturbating"
(1916).

Page 18
Hairy vagina

Page 21
Retro Blow job
retrosex.com

Page 31
Vagina picture

Page 33
Penis Shrine
associated content.com

Page39
Sex horoscopes
Page 42
Anal Sex ad

Page 48
 Group Sex

Miss Mimi's Highly Anticipated Sex Tip Book "Hot Sexy, Dirty, Sex Tips" A *Sexual Self Help Book*. Based on the tips from her #1 rated weekend Gomez Brothers |G-Spot Hour with a worldwide fan base airing exclusively on Shade45/XM66 Saturdays 7pm-8pm est.

Miss Mimi has a collection of "porn star approved" sex tips to spice up your sex life! 10 chapters of HOT *Sexy*, Dirty, *Sexy* TIPS. Miss Mimi outlines and makes the basic moves better and more exciting. This book is based on a survey of 200 sexually active and adventurous couples.
This book is for the Beginner "Self Love is the most important", the Frigid "Tips on how to soothe and encourage an apprehensive lover." and the Super freak " Get Down and Dirty with Miss Mimi's Tips.

"How about a Dick Sandwich with a side of Tossed Salad."

Miss Mimi encourages everyone to
"Nut Up or Shut Up!"

"We all need to be able to express our sexual needs without judgment. I encourage my listeners and readers to ask the tuff sexual questions so they can get to the good part of the relationship!" --Miss MiMi

"Have the Sex you want and Want the Sex you have"-- Miss MiMi

"I love Miss MiMi's sex tips"-- Debbie Dick'em Porn star

MS. MIMI & CO. PUBLISHING

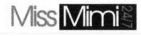

HOT *Sexy, Dirty, Sex* **TIPS** *A sexual Self Help book*